Lean and Green Food

The Complete Cookbook on Lean and Green Diet to Burn Fat and Stay Fit. 50 Healthy and Delicious Recipes to Lose Weight and Regain Your Body Shape with the Fat-Burning Power of these Common Ingredients

By **Sophie Cook**

Table of Contents

Additionally, the information in the following pages is intended only for informational purposes and should thus be thought of as universal. As befitting its nature, it is presented without assurance regarding its prolonged validity or interim quality. Trademarks that are mentioned are done without written consent and can in no way be considered an endorsement from the trademark holder.

Introduction

The Lean and green diet is designed to help people lose weight and fat by reducing calories and carbohydrates through portion-controlled meals and snacks.

Between 6 portioned-controlled meals, the 5&1 plan limits the calories to 800-1,000 calories per day.

A lot of researches also revealed that reducing the total intake of calories is effective for weight loss. The low-carb diets are also included here.

A study was conducted for 16 weeks, having 198 participants with excess weight or obesity. They found out that Lean and Green 5&1 Plan had significantly lower weight, waist circumference, and fat levels than the control group.

The research suggested additional benefits since it resulted in the right way. It associates 5-10 % weight loss with a reduced risk of heart disease and also types two diabetes. Those who also tried the 5&1 Plan lost 5.7% of their body weight, on average, having a percentage of 28.1 % of participants losing over 105.

It is also said that one-on-one coaching is constructive, as well. A similar study was also conducted regarding it. They found out that individuals on the 5&1 diet who have completed at least 75% of the coaching sessions had lost more than twice their original weight, unlike those who only participated in fewer sessions.

All the same, many significant and related studies have also demonstrated and resulted in a substantial improvement with short and long-term weight loss. The diet adherence in programs that includes ongoing coaching is also included in it.

But then, currently, there are no studies yet that have proven the long-term results of the Lean and Green diet. Still, research conducted similar to a diet plan noted that the percentage of participants who have maintained the diet for a year was 25%.

Another research also showed some of them regain weight during the weight maintenance phase while following another diets. Coaching is the only factor that differs from these 5&1 diets and the 5&1 Lean and Green Plan. Overall, it is inevitable that more research is needed to assess the Lean and Green diet's lifetime effectiveness.

The low calorie and low carbohydrates plan of this diet is continuously gathering support from experts since it has been proven to show temporary fat and weight loss. In the future, if more research and study will be done, its long-term effectiveness will now be defined.

The Lean and Green diet is considered a high-protein diet, having a protein that counts up to 10–35% of a person's daily calories. Nevertheless, powdered, processed substances can result in some unpleasant consequences.

According to London, "The additives and protein isolate plus can give you some unnecessary GI side effects that can make an individual feel bloated, making it a lot better with a sugar-free Greek yogurt that contains protein in a smoothie." Also, according to London, "there is no regulation of dietary supplements like powders and shakes for safety by the FDA as there is for foods. Protein blends and powders can contain unwanted ingredients and can interfere with your medication. This makes it important to inform your doctor about what you are trying to indulge yourself in".

Chapter 1. What Is Lean and Green Diet

The Lean and Green Diet encourages people to limit the number of calories that they should take daily. Under this program, dieters are encouraged to consume between 800 and 1000 calories daily. For this to be possible, dieters are encouraged to opt for healthier food items and meal replacements. But unlike other types of commercial diet regimens, the Lean and Green Diet comes in different variations. There are currently three variations of this diet plan that one can choose according to one's needs.

- 5&1 Lean and Green Diet Plan: This is the most common version of this diet, and it involves eating five prepackaged meals from the Optimal Health Fueling and one home-made balanced dinner.

- 4&2&1 Lean and Green Diet Plan: This diet plan is designed for people who want to have flexibility while following this regimen. Under this program, dieters are encouraged to eat more calories and have more flexible food choices. This means that they can consume four prepackaged Optimal Health Fueling food, three home-cooked meals from the Lean and Green, and one snack daily.

- 5&2&2 Lean and Green Diet Plan: This diet plan is perfect for individuals who prefer to have a flexible meal plan to achieve a healthy weight. It is recommended for a wide variety of people. Under this diet regimen, dieters must eat five fueling, two lean and green meals, and two healthy snacks.

- 3&3 Lean and Green Diet Plan: This particular Diet plan is created for people who have moderate weight problems and merely want to maintain a healthy body. Under this diet plan, dieters are encouraged to consume three prepackaged Optimal Health Fuelings and three home-cooked meals.

- Lean and Green for Nursing Mothers: This diet regimen is designed for nursing mothers with babies of at least two months old. Aside from supporting breastfeeding mothers, it also encourages gradual weight loss.

- Lean and Green for Diabetes: This is designed for Type 1 and Type 2 diabetes people. The meal plans are designed to consume more green and lean meals, depending on their needs and condition.

- Lean and Green for Gout: This diet regimen incorporates a balance of low in purines and moderate in protein.

- Lean and Green for seniors (65 years and older): Designed for seniors, this diet plan has some variations following the components of Fuelings depending on the senior dieters' needs and activities.

- Lean and Green for Teen Boys and Teen Girls (13-18 years old): Designed for active teens, this diet for Teen Boys and Teen Girls provides the right nutrition to growing teens.

Regardless of which type of Lean and Green Diet plan you choose, you must talk with a coach to determine which program is right for you based on your individual goals. This is to ensure that you get the most out of the plan that you have chosen.

How to Start This Diet

The Lean and Green Diet is comprised of different phases. A certified coach will educate you on the steps you need to undertake to follow this regimen. But for the sake of those who are new to this diet, below are some of the things that you need to know, especially when you are still starting with this diet regimen.

Initial Steps

During this phase, people are encouraged to consume 800 to 1,000 calories to help them shed off at least 12 pounds within the next 12 weeks. For instance, if you are following the 5&1 Diet Plan, you need to eat a meal every 40 minutes and include a 30-minute moderate workout on most days of your week. You need to consume not more than 100 grams of Carbohydrates daily during this phase.

Further, consuming lean and green meals is highly encouraged. It involves eating 5 to 7 ounces of cooked lean proteins, three servings of non-starchy vegetables, and two healthy fats. This phase also encourages the dieter to include one optional snack per day, such as 1/2 cup sugar-free gelatin, three celery sticks, and 12 ounces nuts. Aside from these things, below are other things that you need to remember when following this phase:

    - Make sure that the portion size recommendations are for cooked weight and not the raw -weight of your ingredients

    - Opt for meals that are baked, grilled, broiled, or poached. Avoid frying foods, as this will increase your calorie intake.

- Eat at least two servings of fish rich in Omega-3 fatty acids. These include fishes like tuna, salmon, trout, mackerel, herring, and other cold-water fishes.
-Choose meatless alternatives like tofu and tempeh.
-Follow the program even when you are dining out. Keep in mind that drinking alcohol is discouraged when following this plan.

Maintenance Phase

As soon as you have achieved your desired weight, the next phase is the transition stage. It is a 6-week stage that involves increasing your calorie intake to 1,550 per day. This is also the phase when you can add more varieties into your meal, such as whole grains, low-fat dairy, and fruits.

After six weeks, you can now move into the 3&3 Lean and Green Diet plan, so you are required to eat three lean and green meals and 3 Fueling foods.

Chapter 2. How It Works

The Lean and Green Diet is viewed as a high-protein diet, with its protein having 10–35% of your daily calories. Be that as it may, the handled, powdered kind can prompt some not exactly beautiful outcomes. "The protein confine in addition to added substances can cause you to feel enlarged and have caused some undesirable GI symptoms, making you off with unsweetened Greek yogurt for protein in a single smoothie," London says.

The FDA also doesn't direct dietary enhancements like shakes and powders for security and viability in a similar way it accomplishes for food. "Powders and protein 'mixes' may have unwanted fixings, or could interface with a drug you might be taking," London includes, "making it extra critical to ensure your doctor knows about you attempting the arrangement." Like many commercial plans, this one involves buying most of the foods permitted on a diet in packaged form. The company deals in a wide range of food products that they call "fuelings"—on its website. These include pancakes, shakes, pasta dishes, soups, cookies, mashed potatoes, and popcorn. Users pick the plan that best suits them. The 5 & 1 Plan entails eating five small meals per day. The meals can be selected from more than 60 substitutable fuelings, including one lean and green meal, probably veggies or protein that you will prepare by yourself. The Optimal Essential Kit, costing $356.15, provides 119 servings, or about 20 days' worth.

A flexible option is the 4 & 2 & 1 Plan. It merely contains four daily fuelings; you can choose and create two of your own lean and green meals and one of the purchased snacks. Also, including a similar mix of convenience food, a kit with 140 servings costs $399.00.

How Much Does Lean and Green Cost?

In comparison, the United States Department of Agriculture estimates that a woman whose ages range from 10-50 can follow a nutritious diet while spending as little as $166.40 per month on groceries. As long as she is preparing all her meals at home.

How Nutritious Is This Diet

Below is the breakdown comparison of meals' nutritional content on the Lean and Green Weight 5&1 Plan and the federal government's 2015 Dietary Guidelines for Americans.

	Optimal Weight 5&1 Plan	**Federal Government Recommendation**
Calories	800-1,000	Men 19-25: 2,800 26-45: 2,600 46-65: 2,400 65+: 2,200 Women 19-25: 2,200 26-50: 2,000 51+: 1,800
Total fat **% of Calorie Intake**	20%	20%-35%

Total Carbohydrates **% of Calorie Intake**	40%	45%-65%
Sugars	10%-20%	N/A
Fiber	25 g – 30 g	Men 19-30: 34 g. 31-50: 31 g. 51+: 28 g. Women 19-30: 28 g. 31-50: 25 g. 51+: 22 g.
Protein	40%	10%-35%
Sodium	Under 2,300 mg	Under 2,300 mg.
Potassium	Average 3,000 mg	At least 4,700 mg.
Calcium	1,000 mg – 1,200 mg	Men 1,000 mg. Women 19-50: 1,000 mg. 51+: 1,200 mg.

Chapter 3.   Breakfast

Coconut Pancakes

Preparation Time: 5 minutes
Cooking Time: 15 minutes
Servings: 4
Ingredients:

- 1 cup coconut flour
- 2 tbsps. arrowroot powder
- 1 tsp. baking powder
- 1 cup coconut milk
- 3 tbsps. coconut oil

Directions:

1. In a medium container, mix in all the dry ingredients.

2. Add the coconut milk and 2 tbsps. of the coconut oil then mix properly.

3. In a skillet, melt 1 tsp. of coconut oil.

4. Pour a ladle of the batter into the skillet then swirl the pan to spread the batter evenly into a smooth pancake.

5. Cook it for like 3 minutes on medium heat until it becomes firm.

6. Turn the pancake to the other side then cook it for another 2 minutes until it turns golden brown.

7. Cook the remaining pancakes in the same process.

8. Serve.

Nutrition:
Calories: 377 kcal
Fat: 14.9g
Carbs: 60.7g
Protein: 6.4g

Whole Grain Bread and Avocado

Preparation Time: 5 minutes
Cooking Time: 0 minutes
Servings: 1
Ingredients:

- 2 slices of wholemeal bread
- 60 g of cottage cheese
- 1 stick of thyme
- ½ avocado
- ½ lime
- Chili flakes
- salt
- pepper

Directions:

1. Cut the avocado in half.

2. Remove the pulp and cut it into slices.

3. Pour the lime juice over it.

4. Wash the thyme and shake it dry.

5. Remove the leaves from the stem.

6. Brush the whole wheat bread with the cottage cheese.

7. Place the avocado slices on top.

8. Top with the chili flakes and thyme.

9. Add salt and pepper and serve.

Nutrition:
kcal: 490
Carbohydrates: 31 g
Protein: 19 g
Fat: 21 g

Crunchy Quinoa Meal

Preparation Time: 5 minutes
Cooking Time: 25 minutes
Servings: 2
Ingredients:

- 3 cups coconut milk
- 1 cup rinsed quinoa
- 1/8 tsp. ground cinnamon
- 1 cup raspberry
- 1/2 cup chopped coconuts

Directions:

1. In a saucepan, pour milk and bring to a boil over moderate heat.

2. Add the quinoa to the milk and then bring it to a boil once more.

3. You then let it simmer for at least 15 minutes on medium heat until the milk is reduced.

4. Stir in the cinnamon then mix properly.

5. Cover it then cook for 8 minutes until the milk is completely absorbed.

6. Add the raspberry and cook the meal for 30 seconds.

7. Serve and enjoy.

Nutrition:
Calories: 271 kcal
Fat: 3.7g
Carbs: 54g
Proteins: 6.5g

Amaranth Porridge

Preparation Time: 5 minutes
Cooking Time: 30 minutes
Servings: 2.
Ingredients:

- 2 cups coconut milk
- 2 cups alkaline water
- 1 cup amaranth
- 2 tbsps. coconut oil
- 1 tbsp. ground cinnamon

Directions:

1. In a saucepan, mix in the milk with water then boil the mixture.

2. You stir in the amaranth then reduce the heat to medium.

3. Cook on the medium heat then simmer for at least 30 minutes as you stir it occasionally.

4. Turn off the heat.

5. Add in cinnamon and coconut oil then stir.

6. Serve.

Nutrition:
Calories: 434 kcal
Fat: 35g
Carbs: 27g
Protein: 6.7g

Chapter 4.   Lunch
Asparagus Frittata Recipe

Preparation Time: 20 minutes
Cooking Time: 20 minutes
Servings: 4
Ingredients:
- Bacon slices, chopped: 4
- Salt and black pepper
- Eggs (whisked): 8
- Asparagus (trimmed and chopped): 1 bunch

Directions:
1. Heat a pan, add bacon, stir and cook for 5 minutes.

2. Add asparagus, salt, and pepper, stir and cook for another 5 minutes.

3. Add the chilled eggs, spread them in the pan, let them stand in the oven and bake for 20 minutes at 350° F.

4. Share and divide between plates and serve for breakfast.

Nutrition:
Calories 251
carbs 16
fat 6
fiber 8
Protein 7

Avocados Stuffed with Salmon

Preparation Time: 5 minutes
Cooking Time: 5 minutes
Servings: 2
Ingredients:

- Avocado (pitted and halved): 1
- Olive oil: 2 tablespoons
- Lemon juice: 1
- Smoked salmon (flaked): 2 ounces
- Goat cheese (crumbled): 1 ounce
- Salt and black pepper

Directions:

1. Combine the salmon with lemon juice, oil, cheese, salt, and pepper in your food processor and pulsate well.

2. Divide this mixture into avocado halves and serve.

3. Dish and Enjoy!

Nutrition:

Calories: 300
Fat: 15
Fiber: 5
Carbs: 8
Protein: 16

Bacon and Brussels Sprout Breakfast

Preparation Time: 10 minutes
Cooking Time: 15 minutes
Servings: 3
Ingredients:

- Apple cider vinegar, 1½ tbsps.
- Salt
- Minced shallots, 2
- Minced garlic cloves, 2
- Medium eggs, 3
- Sliced Brussels sprouts, 12 oz.
- Black pepper
- Chopped bacon, 2 oz.
- Melted butter, 1 tbsp.

Directions:

1. Over medium heat, quick fry the bacon until crispy then reserve on a plate

2. Set the pan on fire again to fry garlic and shallots for 30 seconds

3. Stir in apple cider vinegar, Brussels sprouts, and seasoning to cook for five minutes

4. Add the bacon to cook for five minutes then stir in the butter and set a hole at the center

5. Crash the eggs to the pan and let cook fully

6. Enjoy

Nutrition:
Calories: 275
Fat: 16.5
Fiber: 4.3
Carbs: 17.2
Protein: 17.4

Bacon and Lemon Spiced Muffins

Preparation Time: 10 minutes
Cooking Time: 20 minutes
Servings: 12
Ingredients:

- Lemon thyme, 2 tsps.
- Salt
- Almond flour, 3 cup.
- Melted butter, ½ cup.
- Baking soda, 1 tsp.
- Black pepper
- Medium eggs, 4
- Diced bacon, 1 cup.

Directions:

1. Set a mixing bowl in place and stir in the eggs and baking soda to incorporate well.

2. Whisk in the seasonings, butter, bacon, and lemon thyme

3. Set the mixture in a well-lined muffin pan.

4. Set the oven for 20 minutes at 3500F, allow to bake

5. Allow the muffins to cool before serving

Nutrition:
Calories: 186
Fat: 17.1
Fiber: 0.8
Carbs: 1.8
Protein: 7.4

Chapter 5.   Dinner
Mediterranean Burrito

Preparation Time: 10 minutes
Cooking Time: 0 minutes
Servings: 2
Ingredients:

- 2 wheat tortillas
- 2 oz. red kidney beans, canned, drained
- 2 tablespoons hummus
- 2 teaspoons tahini sauce
- 1 cucumber
- 2 lettuce leaves
- 1 tablespoon lime juice
- 1 teaspoon olive oil
- ½ teaspoon dried oregano

Directions:

1. Mash the red kidney beans until you get a puree.

2. Then spread the wheat tortillas with beans mash from one side.

3. Add hummus and tahini sauce.

4. Cut the cucumber into the wedges and place them over tahini sauce.

5. Then add lettuce leaves.

6. Make the dressing: mix up together olive oil, dried oregano, and lime juice.

7. Drizzle the lettuce leaves with the dressing and wrap the wheat tortillas in the shape of burritos.

Nutrition:
Calories 288
Fat 10.2
Fiber 14.6
Carbs 38.2
Protein 12.5

Sweet Potato Bacon Mash

Preparation Time: 10 minutes
Cooking Time: 20 minutes
Servings: 4
Ingredients:

- 3 sweet potatoes, peeled
- 4 oz. bacon, chopped
- 1 cup chicken stock
- 1 tablespoon butter
- 1 teaspoon salt
- 2 oz. Parmesan, grated

Directions:

1. Chop sweet potato and put it in the pan.

2. Add chicken stock and close the lid.

3. Boil the vegetables for 15 minutes or until they are soft.

4. After this, drain the chicken stock.

5. Mash the sweet potato with the help of the potato masher. Add grated cheese and butter.

6. Mix up together salt and chopped bacon. Fry the mixture until it is crunchy (10-15 minutes).

7. Add cooked bacon in the mashed sweet potato and mix up with the help of the spoon.

8. It is recommended to serve the meal warm or hot.

Nutrition:
Calories 304
Fat 18.1
Fiber 2.9
Carbs 18.8
Protein 17

Prosciutto Wrapped Mozzarella Balls

Preparation Time: 10 minutes
Cooking Time: 10 minutes
Servings: 4
Ingredients:

- 8 Mozzarella balls, cherry size
- 4 oz. bacon, sliced
- ¼ teaspoon ground black pepper
- ¾ teaspoon dried rosemary
- 1 teaspoon butter

Directions:

1. Sprinkle the sliced bacon with ground black pepper and dried rosemary.

2. Wrap every Mozzarella ball in the sliced bacon and secure them with toothpicks.

3. Melt butter.

4. Brush wrapped Mozzarella balls with butter.

5. Line the tray with the baking paper and arrange Mozzarella balls in it.

6. Bake the meal for 10 minutes at 365F.

Nutrition:
Calories 323
Fat 26.8
Fiber 0.1
Carbs 0.6
Protein 20.6

Garlic Chicken Balls

Preparation Time: 15 minutes
Cooking Time: 10 minutes
Servings: 4
Ingredients:

- 2 cups ground chicken
- 1 teaspoon minced garlic
- 1 teaspoon dried dill
- 1/3 carrot, grated
- 1 egg, beaten
- 1 tablespoon olive oil
- ¼ cup coconut flakes
- ½ teaspoon salt

Directions:

1. In the mixing bowl mix up together ground chicken, minced garlic, dried dill, carrot, egg, and salt.

2. Stir the chicken mixture with the help of the fingertips until homogenous.

3. Then make medium balls from the mixture.

4. Coat every chicken ball in coconut flakes.

5. Heat up olive oil in the skillet.

6. Add chicken balls and cook them for 3 minutes from each side. The cooked chicken balls will have a golden-brown color.

Nutrition:
Calories 200
Fat 11.5
Fiber 0.6
Carbs 1.7
Protein 21.9

Chapter 6.   Vegetable

Bell Pepper Eggs

Preparation Time: 10 minutes;
Cooking Time: 4 minutes
Servings: 2
Ingredients

- 1 green bell pepper,
- 2 eggs
- Seasoning:
- 1 tsp coconut oil
- ¼ tsp salt
- ¼ tsp ground black pepper

Directions:

1. Prepare pepper rings, and for this, cut out two slices from the pepper, about ¼-inch, and reserve remaining bell pepper for later use.

2. Take a skillet pan, place it over medium heat, grease it with oil, place pepper rings in it, and then crack an egg into each ring.

3. Season eggs with salt and black pepper, cook for 4 minutes or until eggs have cooked to the desired level.

4. Transfer eggs to a plate and serve.

Nutrition:
110.5 Calories;
8 g Fats;
7.2 g Protein;
1.7 g Net Carb;
1.1 g Fiber;

Omelet-Stuffed Peppers

Preparation Time: 5 minutes
Cooking Time: 20 minutes
Servings: 2
Ingredients

- 1 large green bell pepper, halved, cored
- 2 eggs
- 2 slices of bacon, chopped, cooked
- 2 tbsp. grated parmesan cheese
- Seasoning:
- 1/3 tsp salt
- ¼ tsp ground black pepper

Directions:

1. Turn on the oven, then set it to 400 degrees F, and let preheat.

2. Then take a baking dish, pour in 1 tbsp. water, place bell pepper halved in it, cut-side up, and bake for 5 minutes.

3. Meanwhile, crack eggs in a bowl, add chopped bacon and cheese, season with salt and black pepper, and whisk until combined.

4. After 5 minutes of baking time, remove baking dish from the oven, evenly fill the peppers with egg mixture and continue baking for 15 to 20 minutes until eggs has set.

5. Serve.

Nutrition:
428 Calories;
35.2 g Fats;
23.5 g Protein;
2.8 g Net Carb;
1.5 g Fiber;

Bacon Avocado Bombs

Preparation Time: 10 minutes
Cooking Time: 10 minutes
Servings: 2
Ingredients

- 1 avocado, halved, pitted
- 4 slices of bacon
- 2 tbsp. grated parmesan cheese

Directions:

1. Turn on the oven and broiler and let it preheat.

2. Meanwhile, prepare the avocado and for that, cut it in half, then remove its pit, and then peel the skin.

3. Evenly one half of the avocado with cheese, replace with the other half of avocado and then wrap avocado with bacon slices.

4. Take a baking sheet, line it with aluminum foil, place wrapped avocado on it, and broil for 5 minutes per side, flipping carefully with tong halfway.

5. When done, cut each avocado in half crosswise and serve

Nutrition:
378 Calories;
33.6 g Fats;
15.1 g Protein;
0.5 g Net Carb;
2.3 g Fiber;

Egg in a Hole with Eggplant

Preparation Time: 5 minutes;
Cooking Time: 15 minutes
Servings: 2
Ingredients

- 1 large eggplant
- 2 eggs
- 1 tbsp. coconut oil, melted
- 1 tsp unsalted butter
- 2 tbsp. chopped green onions
- Seasoning:
- ¾ tsp ground black pepper
- ¾ tsp salt

Directions:

1. Set the grill and let it preheat at the high setting.

2. Meanwhile, prepare the eggplant, and for this, cut two slices from eggplant, about 1-inch thick, and reserve the remaining eggplant for later use.

3. Brush slices of eggplant with oil, season with salt on both sides, then place the slices on grill and cook for 3 to 4 minutes per side.

4. Transfer grilled eggplant to a cutting board, let it cool for 5 minutes and then make a home in the center of each slice by using a cookie cutter.

5. Take a frying pan, place it over medium heat, add butter and when it melts, add eggplant slices in it and crack an egg into its each hole.

6. Let the eggs cook for 3 to 4 minutes, then carefully flip the eggplant slice and continue cooking for 3 minutes until the egg has thoroughly cooked.

---

7. Season egg with salt and black pepper, transfer them to a plate, then garnish with green onions and serve.

Nutrition:
184 Calories;
14.1 g Fats;
7.8 g Protein;
3 g Net Carb;
3.5 g Fiber;

Frittata with Spinach and Meat

Preparation Time: 10 minutes;
Cooking Time: 20 minutes
Servings: 2
Ingredients

- 4 oz ground turkey
- 3 oz of spinach leaves
- 1/3 tsp minced garlic
- 1/3 tsp coconut oil
- 2 eggs
- Seasoning:
- 1/3 tsp salt
- ¼ tsp ground black pepper

Directions:

1. Turn on the oven, then set it to 400 degrees F, and let it preheat.

2. Meanwhile, take a skillet pan, place it over medium heat, and add spinach and cook for 3 to 5 minutes until spinach leaves have wilted, remove the pan from heat.

3. Take a small heatproof skillet pan, place it over medium heat, add ground turkey and cook for 5 minutes until thoroughly cooked.

4. Then add spinach, season with salt and black pepper, stir well, then remove the pan from heat and spread the mixture evenly in the pan.

5. Crack eggs in a bowl, season with salt and black pepper, then pour this mixture over spinach mixture in the pan and bake for 10 to 15 minutes until frittata has thoroughly cooked and the top is golden brown.

6. When done, let frittata rest in the pan for 5 minutes, then cut it into slices and serve.

Nutrition:
166 Calories;
13 g Fats;
10 g Protein;
0.5 g Net Carb;
0.5 g Fiber;

Avocado Egg Boat with Cheddar

Preparation Time: 5 minutes
Cooking Time: 15 minutes
Servings: 2
Ingredients

- 1 avocado, halved, pitted
- 2 eggs
- 2 tbsp. chopped bacon
- 2 tbsp. shredded cheddar cheese
- Seasoning:
- 1/8 tsp salt
- 1/8 tsp ground black pepper

Directions:

1. Turn on the oven, then set it to 400 degrees F and let it preheat.

2. Meanwhile, prepare avocado and for this, cut it into half lengthwise and then remove the pit.

3. Scoop out some of the flesh from the center, crack an egg into each half, and then sprinkle with bacon and season with salt and black pepper.

4. Sprinkle cheese over egg and avocado and then bake for 10 to 15 minutes or until the yolk has cooked to desired level.

5. Serve.

Nutrition:
263.5 Calories;
21.4 g Fats;
12 g Protein;
1.3 g Net Carb;
4.6 g Fiber

Chapter 7. Seafood
Foil Packet Salmon

Preparation Time: 5 minutes
Cooking Time: 15 minutes
Servings: 2
Ingredients:
- 2 x 4-oz. skinless salmon fillets
- 2 tbsp. unsalted butter, melted
- ½ tsp. garlic powder
- 1 medium lemon
- ½ tsp. dried dill

Directions:
1. Take a sheet of aluminum foil and cut into two squares measuring roughly 5" x 5". Lay each of the salmon fillets at the center of each piece. Brush both fillets with a tablespoon of bullet and season with a quarter-teaspoon of garlic powder.

2. Halve the lemon and grate the skin of one half over the fish. Cut four half-slices of lemon, using two to top each fillet. Season each fillet with a quarter-teaspoon of dill.

3. Fold the tops and sides of the aluminum foil over the fish to create a kind of packet. Place each one in the fryer.

4. Cook for twelve minutes at 400°F.

5. The salmon is ready when it flakes easily. Serve hot.

Nutrition:
Calories: 240
Fat: 13g
Protein: 21g
Sugar: 9g

Foil Packet Lobster Tail

Preparation Time: 5 minutes
Cooking Time: 15 minutes
Servings: 2
Ingredients:

- 2 x 6-oz. lobster tail halves
- 2 tbsp. salted butter, melted
- ½ medium lemon, juiced
- ½ tsp. Old Bay seasoning
- 1 tsp. dried parsley

Directions:

1. Lay each lobster on a sheet of aluminum foil. Pour a light drizzle of melted butter and lemon juice over each one, and season with Old Bay.

2. Fold down the sides and ends of the foil to seal the lobster. Place each one in the fryer.

3. Cook at 375°F for twelve minutes.

4. Just before serving, top the lobster with dried parsley.

Nutrition:
Calories: 510
Fat: 18g
Protein: 26g
Sugar: 12g

Avocado Shrimp

Preparation Time: 10 minutes
Cooking Time: 20 minutes
Servings: 2
Ingredients:

- ½ cup onion, chopped
- 2 lb. shrimp
- 1 tbsp. seasoned salt
- 1 avocado
- ½ cup pecans, chopped

Directions:

1. Pre-heat the fryer at 400°F.

2. Put the chopped onion in the basket of the fryer and spritz with some cooking spray. Leave to cook for five minutes.

3. Add the shrimp and set the timer for a further five minutes. Sprinkle with some seasoned salt, then allow to cook for an additional five minutes.

4. During these last five minutes, halve your avocado and remove the pit. Cube each half, then scoop out the flesh.

5. Take care when removing the shrimp from the fryer. Place it on a dish and top with the avocado and the chopped pecans.

Nutrition:
Calories: 195
Fat: 14g
Protein: 36g
Sugar: 10g

Lemon Butter Scallops

Preparation Time: 15 minutes
Cooking Time: 30 minutes
Servings: 1
Ingredients:

- 1 lemon
- 1 lb. scallops
- ½ cup butter
- ¼ cup parsley, chopped

Directions:

1. Juice the lemon into a Ziploc bag.

2. Wash your scallops, dry them, and season to taste. Put them in the bag with the lemon juice. Refrigerate for 40 minutes.

3. Remove the bag from the refrigerator and leave for about twenty minutes until it returns to room temperature. Transfer the scallops into a foil pan that is small enough to be placed inside the fryer.

4. Pre-heat the fryer at 400°F and put the rack inside.

5. Place the foil pan on the rack and cook for five minutes.

6. In the meantime, melt the butter in a saucepan over a medium heat. Zest the lemon over the saucepan, then add in the chopped parsley. Mix well.

7. Take care when removing the pan from the fryer. Transfer the contents to a plate and drizzle with the lemon-butter mixture. Serve hot.

Nutrition:
Calories: 420
Fat: 12g
Protein: 23g
Sugar: 13g

Cheesy Lemon Halibut

Preparation Time: 10 minutes
Cooking Time: 20 minutes
Servings: 2
Ingredients:

- 1 lb. halibut fillet
- ½ cup butter
- 2 ½ tbsp. mayonnaise
- 2 ½ tbsp. lemon juice
- ¾ cup parmesan cheese, grated

Directions:

1. Pre-heat your fryer at 375°F.

2. Spritz the halibut fillets with cooking spray and season as desired.

3. Put the halibut in the fryer and cook for twelve minutes.

4. In the meantime, combine the butter, mayonnaise, and lemon juice in a bowl with a hand mixer. Ensure a creamy texture is achieved.

5. Stir in the grated parmesan.

6. When the halibut is ready, open the drawer and spread the butter over the fish with a butter knife. Allow to cook for a further two minutes, then serve hot.

Nutrition:
Calories: 432
Fat: 18g
Protein: 14g
Sugar: 12g

Chapter 8.   Soup and Stew

Okra and Beef Stew

Preparation Time: 15 minutes
Cooking Time: 25 minutes
Servings: 3 servings
Ingredients:

- 6 oz okra, chopped
- 8 oz beef sirloin, chopped
- 1 cup of water
- ¼ cup coconut cream
- 1 teaspoon dried basil
- ¼ teaspoon cumin seeds
- 1 tablespoon avocado oil

Directions:

1. Sprinkle the beef sirloin with cumin seeds and dried basil and put in the instant pot.

2. Add avocado oil and roast the meat on saute mode for 5 minutes. Stir it occasionally.

3. Then add coconut cream, water, and okra.

4. Close the lid and cook the stew on manual mode (high pressure) for 25 minutes. Allow the natural pressure release for 10 minutes.

Nutrition:
calories 216
fat 10.2
Fiber 2.5
Carbs 5.7
Protein 24.6

Chipotle Stew

Preparation Time: 15 minutes
Cooking Time: 10 minutes
Servings: 3 servings
Ingredients:
- 2 chipotle chili in adobo sauce, chopped
- 1 oz. fresh cilantro, chopped
- 9 oz. chicken fillet, chopped
- 1 teaspoon ground paprika
- 2 tablespoons sesame seeds
- ¼ teaspoon salt
- 1 cup chicken broth

Directions:
1. In the mixing bowl mix up chipotle chili, cilantro, chicken fillet, ground paprika, sesame seeds, and salt.

2. Then transfer the Ingredients in the instant pot and add chicken broth.

3. Cook the stew on manual mode (high pressure) for 10 minutes. Allow the natural pressure release for 10 minutes more.

Nutrition:
Calories 230
Fat 10.6
Fiber 2.6
Carbs 4.5
Protein 27.6

Chili

Preparation Time: 10 minutes
Cooking Time: 25 minutes
Servings: 2 servings
Ingredients:

- ½ cup ground beef
- ½ teaspoon chili powder
- 1 teaspoon dried oregano
- ¼ cup crushed tomatoes
- 2 oz. scallions, diced
- 1 teaspoon avocado oil
- ¼ cup of water

Directions:

1. Mix up ground beef, chili powder, dried oregano, and scallions.

2. Then add avocado oil and stir the mixture.

3. Transfer it in the instant pot and cook on saute mode for 10 minutes.

4. Add water and crushed tomatoes. Stir the Ingredients with the help of the spatula until homogenous.

5. Close and seal the lid and cook the chili for 15 minutes on manual mode (high pressure). Then make a quick pressure release.

Nutrition:
Calories 94
Fat 4.6
Fiber 2.4
Carbs 5.6
Protein 8

Pizza Soup

Preparation Time: 10 minutes
Cooking Time: 22 minutes
Servings: 3 servings
Ingredients:

- ¼ cup cremini mushrooms, sliced
- 1 teaspoon tomato paste
- 4 oz. Mozzarella, shredded
- ½ jalapeno pepper, sliced
- ½ teaspoon Italian seasoning
- 1 teaspoon coconut oil
- 5 oz. Italian sausages, chopped
- 1 cup of water

Directions:

1. Melt the coconut oil in the instant pot on saute mode.

2. Add mushrooms and cook them for 10 minutes.

3. After this, add chopped sausages, Italian seasoning, sliced jalapeno, and tomato paste.

4. Mix up the Ingredients well and add water.

5. Close and seal the lid and cook the soup on manual mode (high pressure) for 12 minutes.

6. Then make a quick pressure release and ladle the soup in the bowls. Top it with Mozzarella.

Nutrition:
Calories 289
Fat 23.2
Fiber 0.2
Carbs 2.5
Protein 17.7

Chapter 9.   Sides
Sticky Chicken Thai Wings

Preparation Time: 10 minutes
Cooking Time: 30 minutes
Servings: 6
Ingredients:
- 3 pounds chicken wings removed
- 1 tsp sea salt to taste

For the glaze:
- ¾ cup Thai sweet chili sauce
- ¼ cup soy sauce
- 4 tsp brown sugar
- 4 tsp rice wine vinegar
- 3 tsp fish sauce
- 2 tsp lime juice
- 1 tsp lemon grass minced
- 2 tsp sesame oil
- 1 tsp garlic minced

Directions:
1. Preheat the oven to 350 degrees Fahrenheit. Lightly spray your baking tray with cooking tray and set it aside. To prepare the glaze combine the ingredients in a small bowl and whisk them until they are well combined. Pour half of the mixture into a pan and reserve the rest.

2. Trim any excess skin off the wing edges and season it with pepper and salt. Add the wings to a baking tray and pour the sauce over the wings tossing them for the sauce to evenly coat. Arrange them in a single layer and bake them for 15 minutes.

3. While the wings are in the oven, bring your glaze to simmer in medium heat until there are visible bubbles.

4. Once the wings are cooled on one side rotate each piece and bake for an extra 10 minutes. Baste them and return them into the oven to allow for more cooking until they are golden brown. Garnish with onion slices, cilantro, chili flakes and sprinkle the remain salt. Serving with glaze of your choice.

Nutrition:
Calories: 256
Fat: 16g
Carbohydrates 19g
Proteins: 20g
Potassium: 213mg
Sodium: 561mg

Coconut Shrimp

Preparation Time: 15 minutes
Cooking Time: 15 minutes
Servings: 6
Ingredients:
- Salt and pepper
- 1-pound jumbo shrimp peeled and deveined
- ½ cup all-purpose flour

For batter:
- ½ cup beer
- 1 tsp baking powder
- ½ cup all-purpose flour
- 1 egg

For coating:
- 1 cup panko bread crumbs
- 1 cup shredded coconut

Directions:
1. Line the baking tray with parchment paper.

2. In a shallow bowl add ½ cup flour for dredging and in another bowl whisk the batter ingredients. The batter should resemble a pancake consistency. If it is too thick add a little mineral or beer whisking in between. In another bowl mix together the shredded coconut and bread crumbs.

3. Dredge the shrimp in flour shaking off any excess before dipping in the batter and coat it with bread crumb mixture. Lightly press the coconut into the shrimp.

4. Place them into the baking sheet and repeat the process until you have several.

5. In a Dutch oven skillet heat vegetable oil until it is nice and hot fry the frozen shrimp batches for 3 minutes per side. Drain them on a paper towel lined plate.

6. Serve immediately with sweet chili sauce.

Nutrition:
Calories: 409
Fat 11g
Carbohydrates 46g
Proteins 30g
Sodium: 767mg
Potassium: 345mg

Spicy Korean Cauliflower Bites

Preparation Time: 15 minutes
Cooking Time: 30 minutes
Servings: 4
Ingredients:

- 2 eggs
- 1 lb. cauliflower
- 2/3 cups of corn starch
- 2 tsp smoked paprika
- 1 tsp garlic grated
- 1 tsp ginger grated
- 1 lb. panko
- 1 tsp sea salt

For the Korean barbecue sauce:

- 1 cup ketchup
- ½ cup Korea chili flakes
- ½ cup minced garlic
- ½ cup red pepper

Directions:

1. Cut the cauliflower into small sizes based on your taste and preference.

2. In a small bowl add cornstarch and eggs and mix them until they are smooth.

3. Add onions, garlic, ginger, smoked paprika and coat them with panko.

4. Apply some pressure so that the panko can stick and repeat this with all the cauliflower.

Nutrition:
Calories: 141
Fat: 12 g
Carbs: 23 g
Protein: 27 g

Chapter 10. Desserts
Special Brownies

Preparation Time: 10 minutes
Cooking Time: 22 Minutes
Servings: 4
Ingredients:

- 1 egg
- 1/3 cup cocoa powder
- 1/3 cup sugar
- 7 tbsp. butter
- ½ tbsp. vanilla extract
- ¼ cup white flour
- ¼ cup walnuts
- ½ tbsp. baking powder
- 1 tbsp. peanut butter

Directions:

1. Warm pan with 6 tablespoons butter and the sugar over medium heat, turn, cook for 5 minutes, move to a bowl, put salt, egg, cocoa powder, vanilla extract, walnuts, baking powder and flour, turn mix properly and into a pan.

2. Mix peanut butter with one tablespoon butter in a bowl, heat in microwave for some seconds, turn properly and sprinkle brownies blend over.

3. Put in air fryer and bake at 320° F and bake for 17 minutes.

4. Allow brownies to cool, cut.

5. Serve.

Nutrition:
Calories: 438
Total Fat: 18g
Total carbs: 16.5g

Blueberry Scones

Preparation Time: 10 minutes
Cooking Time: 10 Minutes
Servings: 10
Ingredients:

- 1 cup white flour
- 1 cup blueberries
- 2 eggs
- ½ cup heavy cream
- ½ cup butter
- 5 tbsp. sugar
- 2 tbsp. vanilla extract
- 2 tbsp. baking powder

Directions:

1. Mix in flour, baking powder, salt and blueberries in a bowl and turn.

2. Mix heavy cream with vanilla extract, sugar, butter and eggs and turn properly.

3. Blend the 2 mixtures, squeeze till dough is ready, obtain 10 triangles from mix, put on baking sheet into air fryer and cook them at 320°F for 10 minutes.

4. Serve cold.

Nutrition:
Calories: 525
Total Fat: 21g
Total carbs: 37g

Blueberries Stew

Preparation Time: 10 minutes
Cooking Time: 10 minutes
Servings: 4
Ingredients:

- 2 cups blueberries
- 3 tablespoons stevia
- 1 and ½ cups pure apple juice
- 1 teaspoon vanilla extract

Directions:

1. In a pan, combine the blueberries with stevia and the other ingredients, bring to a simmer and cook over medium-low heat for 10 minutes.

2. Divide into cups and serve cold.

Nutrition:
Calories 192
Fat 5.4
Fiber 3.4
Carbs 9.4
Protein 4.5

Mandarin Cream

Preparation Time: 20 minutes
Cooking Time: 0 minutes
Servings: 8
Ingredients:

- 2 mandarins, peeled and cut into segments
- Juice of 2 mandarins
- 2 tablespoons stevia
- 4 eggs, whisked
- ¾ cup stevia
- ¾ cup almonds, ground

Directions:

1. In a blender, combine the mandarins with the mandarin's juice and the other ingredients, whisk well, divide into cups and keep in the fridge for 20 minutes before serving.

Nutrition:
Calories 106
Fat 3.4
Fiber 0
Carbs 2.4
Protein 4

Chapter 11. Homemade Staples

Chunky Tomato Sauce

Preparation Time: 5 Minutes
Cooking Time: 20 Minutes
Servings: 4
Ingredients:

- 2 tablespoons extra-virgin olive oil
- ½ cup chopped yellow onion (about ½ a medium onion)
- 1 (28-ounce) can diced tomatoes
- 2 tablespoons tomato paste
- 2 garlic cloves, minced
- 1 teaspoon dried basil
- ½ teaspoon dried oregano
- Salt
- Freshly ground black pepper

Directions:

1. In a medium sauce pot, heat the olive oil over medium heat and add the onion. Sauté for 3 minutes. Add the tomatoes and their juices, tomato paste, garlic, basil, and oregano. Stir to combine and let simmer for 15 minutes. Season with salt and pepper.

2. Store in an airtight container in the refrigerator for up to 2 weeks.

3. Freeze Allow the sauce to completely cool, then store in a freezer-safe container for up to 3 months.

Nutrition:
Calories: 111
Fat: 8g
Protein: 2g
Total Carbs: 11g
Fiber: 3g
Sodium: 57mg
Iron: 1mg

Sun-Dried Tomato Tapenade

Preparation Time: 5 Minutes
Cooking Time: 0 Minutes
Servings: 1
Ingredients:
- ½ cup pitted kalamata olives
- ½ cup oil-packed sun-dried tomatoes
- ¼ cup tightly packed fresh basil
- ¼ cup tightly packed fresh parsley

Directions:
1. In a food processor, combine the olives, sun-dried tomatoes, basil, and parsley and pulse to mix. Scrape down the sides of the bowl and continue processing until a semi-smooth paste forms.

2. Store in an airtight container in the refrigerator for up to 1 week.

3. Freeze Store in a freezer-safe container for up to 3 months. To thaw, refrigerate overnight.

Nutrition:
Calories: 16
Fat: 1g
Protein: 0g
Total Carbs: 2g
Fiber: 0g
Sodium: 63mg
Iron: 0mg

Peanut Sauce for Everything

Preparation Time: 5 Minutes
Cooking Time: 0 Minutes
Servings: 1
Ingredients:

- ¼ cup peanut butter
- 3 tablespoons water, plus more to thin
- 2 tablespoons soy sauce (or tamari for gluten-free)
- 2 teaspoons sesame oil
- Juice of 1 lime
- ½ teaspoon sriracha

Directions:

1. Into a blender, drop the peanut butter, water, soy sauce, sesame oil, lime juice, and sriracha. Process until smooth, adding additional water to thin to your desired consistency.

2. Store in an airtight container in the refrigerator for up to 3 days.

Nutrition:
Calories: 122
Fat: 10g
Protein: 5g
Total Carbs: 5g
Fiber: 1g
Sodium: 530mg
Iron: 2mg

Lemon Arugula Pesto

Preparation Time: 5 Minutes
Cooking Time: 0 Minutes
Servings: 1
Ingredients:

- 2 cups fresh baby arugula
- ½ cup grated Parmesan cheese
- 3 tablespoons raw, unsalted walnuts
- 2 garlic cloves, chopped
- ½ teaspoon salt
- ½ cup plus 1 tablespoon extra-virgin olive oil
- Juice of ½ lemon

Directions:

1. In a food processor, combine the arugula, Parmesan, walnuts, garlic, and salt. Process on high for 30 seconds. Add the olive oil and lemon juice and continue to process on high, stopping as needed to scrape down the sides of the bowl, until the mixture is blended smooth.

2. Store in an airtight container in the refrigerator for up to 1 week.

3. Freeze Pesto can be frozen in an airtight, freezer-safe container, or divided into ice cube trays to form cubes, for up to 1 month. To thaw, refrigerate overnight.

Nutrition:
Calories: 157
Fat: 16g
Protein: 3g
Total Carbs: 1g
Fiber: 0g
Sodium: 215mg
Iron: 0mg

Chapter 12.   Poultry

Chicken Fillets with Artichoke Hearts

Preparation Time: 10 minutes
Cooking Time: 30 minutes
Servings: 3
Ingredients:

- 1 can artichoke hearts, chopped
- 12 oz. chicken fillets (3 oz. each fillet)
- 1 teaspoon avocado oil
- ½ teaspoon ground thyme
- ½ teaspoon white pepper
- 1/3 cup water
- 1/3 cup shallot, roughly chopped
- 1 lemon, sliced

Directions:

1. Mix up together chicken fillets, artichoke hearts, avocado oil, ground thyme, white pepper, and shallot.

2. Line the baking tray with baking paper and place the chicken fillet mixture in it.

3. Then add sliced lemon and water.

4. Bake the meal for 30 minutes at 375F. Stir the ingredients during cooking to avoid burning.

Nutrition:
Calories 267,
Fat 8.2 g,
Fiber 3.8 g,
Carbs 10.4 g,
Protein 35.2 g

Chicken Loaf

Preparation Time: 10 minutes
Cooking Time: 40 minutes
Servings: 4
Ingredients:

- 2 cups ground chicken
- 1 egg, beaten
- 1 tablespoon fresh dill, chopped
- 1 garlic clove, chopped
- ½ teaspoon salt
- 1 teaspoon chili flakes
- 1 onion, minced

Directions:

1. In the mixing bowl combine together all ingredient and mix up until you get smooth mass.

2. Then line the loaf dish with baking paper and put the ground chicken mixture inside.

3. Flatten the surface well.

4. Bake the chicken loaf for 40 minutes at 355F.

5. Then chill the chicken loaf to the room temperature and remove from the loaf dish.

6. Slice it.

Nutrition:

Calories 167,
Fat 6.2 g,
Fiber 0.8 g,
Carbs 3.4 g,
Protein 32.2 g

Chicken Meatballs with Carrot

Preparation Time: 10 minutes
Cooking Time: 10 minutes
Servings: 8
Ingredients:
- 1/3 cup carrot, grated
- 1 onion, diced
- 2 cups ground chicken
- 1 tablespoon semolina
- 1 egg, beaten
- ½ teaspoon salt
- 1 teaspoon dried oregano
- 1 teaspoon dried cilantro
- 1 teaspoon chili flakes
- 1 tablespoon coconut oil

Directions:
1. In the mixing bowl combine together grated carrot, diced onion, ground chicken, semolina, egg, salt, dried oregano, cilantro, and chili flakes.

2. With the help of scooper make the meatballs.

3. Heat up the coconut oil in the skillet.

4. When it starts to shimmer, put meatballs in it.

5. Cook the meatballs for 5 minutes from each side over the medium-low heat.

Nutrition:
Calories 107,
Fat 4.2 g,
Fiber 0.8 g,
Carbs 2.4 g,
Protein 11.2 g

Chicken Burgers

Preparation Time: 15 minutes
Cooking Time: 15 minutes
Servings: 4
Ingredients:

- 8 oz. ground chicken
- 1 cup fresh spinach, blended
- 1 teaspoon minced onion
- ½ teaspoon salt
- 1 red bell pepper, grinded
- 1 egg, beaten
- 1 teaspoon ground black pepper
- 4 tablespoons Panko breadcrumbs

Directions:

1. In the mixing bowl mix up together ground chicken, blended spinach, minced garlic, salt, grinded bell pepper, egg, and ground black pepper.

2. When the chicken mixture is smooth, make 4 burgers from it and coat them in Panko breadcrumbs.

3. Place the burgers in the non-sticky baking dish or line the baking tray with baking paper.

4. Bake the burgers for 15 minutes at 365F.

5. Flip the chicken burgers on another side after 7 minutes of cooking.

Nutrition:
Calories 177,
Fat 5.2 g,
Fiber 1.8 g,
Carbs 10.4 g,
Protein 13.2 g

Chapter 13. Fast and Cheap

Beet Salad (From Israel)

Preparation Time: 5 minutes
Cooking Time: 0 minutes
Servings: 2
Ingredients:

- 2–3 fresh, raw beets grated or shredded in food processor
- 3 tablespoons olive oil
- 2 tablespoons balsamic vinegar
- ¼ teaspoon salt
- 1/3 teaspoon cumin
- Dash stevia powder or liquid
- Dash pepper

Directions:

1. Mix all ingredients together for the best raw beet salad.

Nutrition:
Calories: 156
Protein: 8g
Carbohydrate: 40g
Fat: 5 g

Broccoli Salad

Preparation Time: 5 minutes
Cooking Time: 0 minutes
Servings: 2
Ingredients:
- 1 head broccoli, chopped
- 2–3 slices of fried bacon, crumbled
- 1 diced green onion
- ½ cup raisins or craisins
- ½–1 cup of chopped pecans
- ¾ cup sunflower seeds
- ½ cup of pomegranate

Dressing:
- 1 cup organic mayonnaise
- ¼ cup baking stevia
- 2 teaspoons white vinegar

Directions:
1. Mix all ingredients together. Mix dressing and fold into salad.

Nutrition:
Calories: 239
Protein: 10g
Carbohydrate: 33g
Fat: 2 g

Rosemary Garlic Potatoes

Preparation Time: 5 minutes
Cooking Time: 30 minutes
Servings: 2
Ingredients:

- 5 red new potatoes, chopped
- ¼ cup olive oil
- 2–3 cloves of minced garlic
- 1 tablespoon rosemary

Directions:

1. Preheat oven to 425 degrees.

2. Stir all ingredients together in a bowl. Pour onto a baking sheet and bake for 30 minutes.

Nutrition:
Calories: 176
Protein: 5g
Carbohydrate: 30g
Fat: 2 g

Chapter 14. Bread

No Corn Cornbread

Preparation Time: 10 minutes
Cooking Time: 20 minutes
Servings: 8
Ingredients

- ½ cup almond flour
- ¼ cup coconut flour
- ¼ tsp. salt
- ¼ tsp. baking soda
- 3 eggs
- ¼ cup unsalted butter
- 2 tbsp. low-carb sweetener
- ½ cup coconut milk

Directions

1. Preheat the oven to 325F. Line a baking pan.

2. Mix all the dry ingredients in a bowl.

3. Add all the wet ingredients to the dry ones and blend well.

4. Pour the batter into the baking pan and bake for 20 minutes.

5. Cool, slice, and serve.

Nutrition

Calories: 65
Fat: 6g
Carb: 2g
Protein: 2g

Double Chocolate Zucchini Bread

Preparation Time: 10 minutes
Cooking Time: 35 minutes
Servings: 12
Ingredients
- ½ cup coconut flour
- ½ cup chocolate chips (sugar free)
- 2 cups zucchini (shredded)
- 1 tsp. vanilla
- 4 large eggs
- ¼ cup coconut oil, melted
- ¼ tsp. salt
- 1 tsp. baking powder
- 1 tsp. baking soda
- ½ tsp. ground cinnamon
- ½ cup low carb sweetener
- ½ cup cocoa powder (unsweetened)

Directions
1. In a bowl, combine coconut flour, salt, baking powder, cinnamon, sweetener, baking soda, and cocoa.

2. Blend in the vanilla, coconut oil, and eggs. Mix well.

3. Fold in the chocolate chips and zucchini.

4. Line a loaf pan (9 x 5) with parchment paper and pour the mixture in it.

5. Bake at 350F for 40 minutes.

6. Remove from the oven and cool.

7. Serve.

Nutrition
Calories: 124
Fat: 10g
Carb: 7g
Protein: 4g

Blueberry Bread

Preparation Time: 15 minutes
Cooking Time: 40 minutes
Servings: 12
Ingredients

- 10 tbsp. coconut flour
- 1 ½ tsp. baking powder
- ½ tsp. salt
- 2 tbsp. heavy whipping cream
- 1 ½ tsp. vanilla
- 2/3 cup Monkfruit classic
- 2 tbsp. sour cream
- ½ tsp. cinnamon
- ¾ cup fresh blueberries
- 9 tbsp. melted butter
- 6 eggs

For the icing

- ¼ tsp. lemon zest
- 1 tbsp. heavy whipping cream
- dash of vanilla
- 1 tsp. butter (melted)
- 2 tbsp. Monkfruit powdered

Directions

1. Line a regular loaf pan with parchment paper and preheat oven to 350F.

2. Melt butter.

3. Beat eggs, cinnamon, baking powder, salt, vanilla, whipping cream, sour cream, and Monkfruit until combined.

4. Add melted butter and mix well.

5. Add coconut flour and mix well.

6. Add a small amount of batter in the loaf pan and sprinkle with a couple of blueberries. Then spread more batter and sprinkle blueberries on top. Repeat to finish the batter and blueberries.

7. Bake for 65 to 75 minutes. Cool.

8. For the icing, combine all ingredients and whisk.

9. Drizzle over warm bread and serve.

Nutrition
Calories: 155
Fat: 13g
Carb: 4g
Protein: 3g

Fluffy Chaffle

Preparation Time: 3 min
Cooking Time: 4 min
Servings: 1
Ingredients

- 1 egg
- 1/2 cup cheddar cheese, shredded

Directions:

1. Switch on the waffle maker according to manufacturer's instructions

2. Crack egg and combine with cheddar cheese in a small bowl

3. Place half batter on waffle maker and spread evenly.

4. Cook for 4 minutes or until as desired

5. Gently remove from waffle maker and set aside for 2 minutes so it cools down and become crispy

6. Repeat for remaining batter

7. Serve with desired toppings

Nutrition:
Calories: 363
Protein: 2
Fat: 40
Carbohydrates: 1

Chapter 15. Conclusion

Thank you for making it to the end. The Lean and Green Diet can be effectively used for rapid weight loss compared to other plans simply because of the offer made by lean and green meals and its few calories.

This diet depends on strongly confining calories to advance weight reduction. Most "fuelings" drift around 100–110 calories each, which means you could take in about 1,000 calories for every day on this diet.

London concurs that there's a unique way to deal with enduring weight reduction: '"Eating dinners and tidbits that join heaps of produce, 100% entire grains, nuts, seeds, vegetables, and heartbeats, low-Fat: dairy items, eggs, poultry, fish, and lean hamburger in addition to certain extravagances is the most ideal approach to get more fit economically for the long stretch."

You should avoid refined grain, sugar-improved beverages, singed food, and alcohol on the Lean and Green Diet when doing it. During the advancement and upkeep organizes, some carb-containing nourishments are incorporated back in, for instance, low Fat: dairy and new natural products.

The coaching component can be compared to Jenny Craig and Weight Watchers, which urge users to register for meet-ups to get the necessary support. Due to the highly processed nature of the majority of foods available on the Lean and Green Diet, it could pose a threat or challenge compared to the variety of whole, fresh foods you can consume on more self-sustainable plans such as Atkins.

This revolutionary diet enables weight loss through one-on-one coaching, low-carb homemade meals, and low-calorie prepackaged diets. Although the initial 5&1 Plan is quite limiting, the 3&3 maintenance phase enables fewer processed snacks and a wider variety of food, making it easier to lose weight and adhere to the program for sustenance in the long term.

Nevertheless extended calorie restriction may lead to nutrient deficiencies and other risky health concerns.

Although the program promotes Fat: loss and short-term weight loss, further research is required to evaluate the level of lifestyle changes it needs for long-term success.

The bottom line:

The "Lean and Green" weight loss plan promotes weight loss via low-calorie prepackaged meals; quiet carb homemade food, and personalized coaching.

The Lean and Green diet advances weight reduction using low-calorie prepackaged foods, low carb natively constructed suppers, and customized instruction.

However the diet is repetitive and doesn't accommodate all nutritional wishes. What's extra, extended calorie limit may also result in nutrient deficiencies and different potential health issues.

Simultaneously, as this system promotes quick-time period weight and Fat's loss, similarly research is wanted to assess whether it encourages the everlasting way of life adjustments needed for long-time period achievement.

I hope you have learned something!